Simple steps to health and fitness

How to get fit from the comfort of your home for free..

By Rob James

Table of Contents

Dedication

Thank you to my Wife you know who you are for the patience in waiting for this to be published.

Images used under license from Shutterstock

Introduction

DISCOVER: How Simple Steps can Get you fit and healthy and <u>Stop Feeling Overwhelmed</u> by endless fitness and dieting information.

Don't like how your body looks or feel ashamed when you go swimming? Tired of feeling tired and unfit? Or are you just looking for a simple low cost way to get fit and healthy?

All these challenges are covered in the book: *Simple steps to health and fitness*

About Simple steps to health and fitness.

Rob James will show you how to take steps to simplify your diet manage and keep your motivation to exercise, and undertake quick and easy bodyweight exercises to reach your fitness goals.

This book is written for the person who would like to get fit, has tried but failed at different diets or workout routines and would like a more simple way to get fit and healthy without expensive gym fees. It's for the beginner or more experienced person who would like to improve their motivation and fitness routines. Not only will you learn simple fitness and health tips that you can undertake any time and where, you'll also learn routines for beginners intermediate and higher fitness levels as you progress.

If you have a desire get fit and healthy, simplify workout routines -- and save on money spent on gym fees or equipment -- then download today.

Why YOU Should Check Simple steps to health and fitness.

This book will be a good fit if you:
- **Feel overwhelmed by the sheer volume of fitness and health information available online and in magazines**
-
- Struggle to find the time or space to workout

- **Have little time to work out or get to them gym**

- Feel self conscious or embarrassed about going to the gym and feeling people are looking at you.

- **Find yourself confused by all the different workout routines there are available.**

- Tired of paying expensive gym fees or feeling guilty about not getting to the gym enough.

- **Would like to improve your motivation and set specific goals around your health and fitness.**

- Concerned that your partner, friends or strangers are looking at your weight, diet or fitness.

- **Just want to get fit and healthy as easily, simply and low cost as possible**

Want solutions to all of the above?

If you have a desire to get fit and healthy -- and improve your motivation to do all this -- then you should check out Simple steps to health and fitness.

Take action now! Pick up your copy today by clicking the *Buy Now* button at the top of this page

Chapter 1

Starting Strong

There are many different reasons why a person decides to get fit. Have you ever thought of 'why' you want to get fit or lose weight? Is it to look good? To fit into your clothes better? To feel more energetic? To improve your health or reduce risk of ill health? In this chapter, we'll talk about what would make you start and what would keep you going.

Setting Yourself for Success

When it comes to health and fitness, we are only given two options: to take care of ourselves or just allow time to take its toll. If you want to choose the former, then congratulations! The decision of choosing to be fit and healthy is actually the first step to a higher-quality of life.

The decision to be healthier is one thing but the execution is another. What's next and where do you start? The answer is simple: a proper diet and exercise. Those who choose to really do something about their health are people who watch the quality and the quantity of their diet and exercise regularly. On a daily basis, they feel energized and good all day, less stressed, more confident and physically, mentally and even emotionally stronger. In the long run, they have greater chance to avoid chronic diseases like heart attack, stroke, diabetes, osteoporosis etc. and even live a longer life than those who choose to let time and bad habits take their toll on their bodies.

Choosing to be fit and healthy should be a lifestyle change, something that you can do for the rest of your life. Before you undergo a major shift, setting yourself for success is the most important stage. You have to build the right motivation to ensure that you follow through and stick to it until it becomes second nature. Here are some steps to start strong and stay motivated to a healthier life.

Setting Clear Goals

To properly fuel your motivation, the first thing that you should do is set clear goals. This will give you an exact beginning; the feeling of really doing it. Also, this will allow you to work in accordance with your goal and have concrete actions to work efficiently towards it.

Now, ask yourself, what is your goal? If you answered "to get fitness", that is acceptable, but this is too general. This can be your overall, long term goal. How do you achieve it?

You should break down your overall goal into smaller ones that should be **s**pecific, **m**easurable, **a**ttainable, **r**easonable, and **t**ime-based, in other words, **SMART**. The more , Specific, Measurable, achievable, Realistic and time-bound your goals are, you'll work more efficiently and have more chances of success. Based on these criteria, when making goals and planning how to achieve them, write down your answers to these "W" questions.

1. What specific thing do you want to achieve?
2. When do intend to finish this goal?
3. Why do you want to do this?
4. How do you intend to reach the goal (specific actions to take)?

Sample answer:
- Goal: Lose 3kg
- When: In 2 months
- Why: Because I want to fit into my old clothes and feel better about my body
- How: Measure my weight before I start, do bodyweight exercises for 4-5 days a week, east less sugary snacks and eat more vegetables.

General goals that people usually make are statements like "I want to lose weight", "I want to get in shape", and "I want to look better". You can start with this and make small, specific goals like the one above and concentrate on working towards them. Work within your timetable and the ways that you have listed to achieve them.

List all your small goals that coincide with your overall goal and even add new ones as you progress. Place your 'goal list' in places where you'll always see it; on your phone, purse/wallet or laptop, to constantly remind you of what you're working towards.

Remember, baby steps, small achievements, and tiny improvements all add up to larger successes and sustainable changes. Even small set backs on the way are not to be feared but embraced as ongoing signs that you are changing and your old bad habits are just trying to make a last ditch attempt to get you to go back to they way you used to be.

Even if you have small lapses, eating fast food, remember that it is the overall trend that will get you to your goal. So keep to a healthy diet, regular exercise and keep focused on your goal.

Proper and Positive Mindset

In getting fit and being healthy you're not only training your body; you're also training your mind. Your motivation comes from the how you view things as they are happening. Having a proper and positive mindset towards fitness and health will go a long way. Conversely of course a negative mindset will undermine all your work as it will sap your motivation and destroy your confidence.

Eliminate Excuses

Excuses. They are the things that are made by your mind to choose comfort over effort.

In your journey to a fit and healthy body, good habits and some sacrifices are important. You don't get a fit body by skipping exercise and being careful what and when you eat. You have to work for your goals; day after day you have to keep them in mind. These sacrifices, however, are not that big when you come to think of it. In simple steps to fitness and health, time shouldn't be a problem and equipment shouldn't be a problem. In fact, the only thing that keeps you from doing your exercises and eating well is you. You should learn to think of your goals first and set aside the perceived comfort that fuels all the excuses you may have or might make.

Every time you're thinking of skipping exercise, ask yourself, what's more important, your goals or the temporary comfort of not exercising When you look at it this way, it's just between a small amount of effort versus the short-term pleasure of not doing it; a matter of deciding to start or not. Your excuses are often the main culprits that hinder you on doing your exercises, and actually they are all in your mind. So, how do we eliminate these and make sure you get your butt off your comfort zone and start getting fitter?

First, list down all the excuses that you make. What do you usually say to yourself when you're thinking about skipping exercising? Here are the common excuses that people make:

- I'm too tired.
- I don't have enough time./ I'm too busy.
- I don't feel well.
- I have children. Working out is impossible for me.
- I don't know how to exercise/workout.
- I don't have someone I can do it with.

Next, beside these excuses, list the possible ways or reasons to counteract the excuse. Here are some examples on how to beat the common workout excuses that people make.

- I'm too tired.
    - o You'll feel less tired when and after you exercise. People usually feel energetic, even in a good mood, after working out because of the endorphins that the body releases during the process.
    - o You can just do it for a few minutes and if you still feel tired, stop.
    - o Identify the time of the day when you feel energetic and adjust your schedule to squeeze in some exercise/workouts.
- I don't have enough time.
    - o When you make your fitness and health goals one of your top priorities, you will find time to do them.
    - o You can do shorter yet intense workouts to maximize efficiency and efficacy.

- Find the time of the day or the week when you are less busy. Once you note them, take out your organizer and schedule your short workouts.
- Fit exercise into any free time, walking to the bus/station instead of driving, do short exercises in between adverts on the tv.

- I have children to take care of.
  - In working out, especially bodyweight exercises, your imagination is the limit. Find ways to work out while taking care of them.
  - Working out can even be included in your bonding time. You can do bodyweight exercises while having your kids ride your back (make sure you can carry their weight to avoid injuries) or play Frisbee or football in a park.
- I don't feel well
  - Be critical with yourself if you catch yourself making excuses or over playing an injury. Can you do alternative exercise i.e. walking that would not add any stress to an injury?
  - If you're really sick, though, it's not recommended to work your body very hard. However, there are still some things that you can do to stay active while not feeling well. You can try simple stretching or breathing exercises.
- I don't know how to train.
  - Information can come as fast as a click of computer mouse. If you can't find someone to teach you how to properly train, the internet contains almost everything that you need to know. And of course now you have this book.
  - All you need is determination.
- I don't have a workout buddy.
  - Your goals are yours and only you can achieve them. Not having a workout buddy is not an excuse to not exercise.
  - In fact, some experts believe that having a workout buddy is counterproductive. For example, when your workout buddy decides that he/she is too lazy to exercise, you're most likely to feel the same.

Make exercise a habit. Incorporate it into your daily routine. Get rid of all the mental hindrances, also known as, excuses.

Invision your Success

You are what you think. If you see yourself succeeding, you eventually will. Claim and believe that you will achieve your fitness goals and you will reach them. It might take time but with a clear focus on them you will get there.

Start by looking up what physical and body image goals you want to achieve. You can look up pictures of the dream body that you want (make sure that you are making realistic assumptions) and use these as a motivation to exercise every day. Envision yourself having that ideal body that you want while doing exercises that you enjoy doing. Imagine not having to dread your exercise or workouts because you genuinely love doing them and the only thing that you wouldn't want is to let a day pass without doing them.

Picture yourself feeling better, fitter and healthier. Your joints are not hurting, you're not out of breath when you climb up the stairs and you dont have problems keeping up your energy levels or with your children's energy if you have them.

Envision yourself succeeding because you will.

Have Positive Affirmations

Sometimes, all the motivation that you need is in the form of words and thoughts. Positive affirmations (talking to yourself positively) are essential in setting a proper mindset when it comes to changing your mindset and in this case getting and staying fit. Your attitude towards your exercises and how it affects you physically, mentally and emotionally, are important in making you strong in every aspect of your health and your life.

Positive affirmations will serve as your guide and these thoughts will channel your positive energy and focus on achieving your goals. Feed your mind with self-supporting and encouraging words. A healthy and focused mind will eventually result in a healthier body.

You might of course like I did at the beginning think this is all hocus pocus psychobabble. But do you remember what you felt like when someone encouraged you or gave you a compliment? You probably got a short boost of energy, confidence and possibly even happiness. Unfortunately it isnt posible to have that sort of feedback all the time unless of course you do it for yourself. Encouraging yourself and praising success can play a big part in keeping you going. Ok yes, you may look a little crazy talking to yourself in the mirror or when out doing exercises but remember you are doing what you are doing for your goals and not for what other people may think of you.

Here are some positive affirmations that you can practice for these common situations. Of course you can adapt them to your pariticular goals for style.

When you don't feel like working out:

1. I am happy before, during and after I work out.
2. Working out daily makes me feel like a superstar!
3. My mood booster is exercise.

4. Every time I work out, I get closer and closer to my goals.
5. Finding time to work out is natural and easy for me.

When you feel like you can't do it:
1. I will surpass this and I will emerge stronger.
2. I am living a healthier life.
3. I am on my way to a healthy and fit lifestyle and I will never give up.
4. I can feel my body changing for the better.
5. I love the feeling of being fit and I will continue to do things that are geared towards my goals.

When you feel like giving up:
1. Every day I feel better! Every day I am improving!
2. I have come far and I can go farther.
3. I'm pushing myself to the maximum and I'm more encouraged than ever.
4. I will be the strongest, healthiest and happiest version of me.
5. I can do it! I can! I definitely can and I will!

When you're working out:
1. I am doing my exercise with intensity.
2. My energy level is very high and I love it!
3. The pain from my workouts is worth it. I am taking care of myself well.
4. My body feels light, my heart is beating strong and my lungs are working.
5. I can feel my energy levels surging.

Monitoring your Progress

The next step to fueling your motivation is making sure that you monitor your progress. By checking the changes in your body, the way you feel and your overall fitness, you'll find motivation in your improvements and get pumped up into doing more.
Here are some ways to effectively monitor your progress:

NUMERICAL MEASUREMENTS

- There are different kinds of measurements that you can take before you start. These numerical measurements can help you track your progress but you shouldn't restrict yourself to only one kind of measurement.
- Also, when monitoring the changes, make sure that you don't do it on a daily basis. Measure after 1-2 weeks after your recent measurements.

a. Weight
o *Equipment: Scale*

- The most convenient (yet not very accurate) way of measuring your progress is measuring your weight. A scale is very easy to obtain and they are virtually available anywhere.
- As an initial step in your fitness journey, weigh yourself accordingly.
- If your goal is to lose weight, checking your weight every two weeks and seeing those numbers go down can probably be a good indication that you really are losing all the unwanted fat.
- However, if you are also aiming to build muscle, the scale can't accurately discern if you are gaining muscle or fat.
- Beware! Do not obsessively weigh yourself and on a daily basis. Your weight is affected by so many factors like hormones (especially for certain points in a woman's cycle), water retention, time of the day, food and water intake and many more and it fluctuates every day.

b. Body measurements

- *Equipment: Tape measure*
- Another addition to the convenient ways to measure your progress is through taking body measurements and vital statistics.
  - *Neck*: Take the tape around your neck and measure the circumference
  - *Shoulders*: Pin your arms to your side and have someone measure you from shoulder to shoulder
  - *Chest:* Measure the circumference by taking the tape around your chest, placing it just above your nipples, and taking the measurement after putting your arms back down
  - *Biceps*: Measure the widest circumference. You can choose the right or the left arm and use that same arm for the next
  - *Forearms*: Measure the widest circumference. Be consistent if you're using the left or the right.
  - *Waist*: Measure at the narrowest point of your waist. It's usually just above your navel.
  - *Hips*: Measure the widest circumference. It's usually the widest part of your hipbones.
  - *Legs*: While standing, measure the widest circumference. Make sure that you remember where exactly you measured.

c. Body Mass Index (BMI)

- *Equipment: Scale, Height Measuring tape, BMI calculator (online)*
- The Body Mass Index is an estimate of the percentage of your body fat in relation to your height and weight. It gives you an idea if you have a healthy weight, or if you're underweight, overweight or obese.
- To know your BMI, you have to measure your weight and height. There are online calculators that you can easily use to know if your BMI is normal.

o Your BMI should be around 18.5-24.9 for your weight to be considered normal. Numbers higher than these can indicate that you are overweight and if it reaches 30 and above, you are already considered obese.

d. Body Fat Percentage
o *Equipment: Skin Fold Caliper*
o In measuring your body fat percentage by using a caliper, you are measuring the thickness of the skinfold at certain points of your body. The general idea is the thicker the skinfold, the higher the fat on that point.
o To measure the skinfold, do the 'pinch-and-pull'. Pinch the site and pull it to separate the fat tissue.
o Taking this idea into consideration, there are actually two ways to compute for your body fat percentage: the three-site method and the seven-site method.
o The easiest and most reproducible test is the **three-site method**.
- Before measuring, get a marker to lightly mark the spot where you'll measure and take a picture of it. This will help you remember the exact point for future measurements.
- For men, usual sites where you can pinch and pull include the chest (pinch a vertical fold at the point between your armpit and nipple), the abdomen (pinch a vertical fold one inch on one side, right or left, of your navel), and thigh (pinch a vertical fold at the middle point from your hip to your knee).
- For women, usual sites where you can pinch and pull include the triceps (pinch a vertical fold at the midpoint between the bony tip of your shoulder to your elbow), top of your hipbone (pinch a diagonal fold just above the bone of your hip) and thigh (pinch a vertical fold at the middle point from your hip to your knee).
- To compute for your body fat percentage, just search for an online body fat percentage calculator (which saves a lot of time and effort) where you can simply input all three measurements.
o Measure and calculate your body fat percentage every week or every two weeks.

NON-NUMERICAL MONITORING

Of course, your progress should not only be limited to numbers. You also have to consider the overall effects of your fitness regimen.
e. Journaling
o Write everything out. Have a fitness journal where you'll write all your numerical and non-numerical measurements.
o You might opt to divide this into two sections (numerical and non-numerical) to avoid mixing up and confusion.

- In the non-numerical part, write all the things that you feel in all aspects of your fitness journey. Journal how you feel after skipping an exercise, how you feel after a day of overeating, how you feel after a workout, after eating a healthy meal, after checking your body fat percentage go down etc.
- By writing everything down, you might find patterns in your behavior that you wouldn't usually notice. You should also note that your feelings should not dictate whether you work out or not but that your goals dictate what you do.

f. Proof of improved fitness
- One of the other ways to measure how far you've gone is actually realizing how differently you feel after some time of working out.
- Notice how you can do things that you thought you couldn't do before you started. For me this was running for the bus, now I can do it without having a heart attack in the process.
- Identify your little successes: not feeling out of breath after climbing a flight of stairs, running for a bus, being able to lift the shopping into the car with ease, being able to refuse a cake or sweet treat, finally keeping up with your children's energy, not feeling groggy in the office, etc.

g. The mirror
- Looking at a mirror, you will notice a lot of changes.
- You can find differences in your body, like how the skin on your triceps used to sag but now is less jiggly, how your legs look more toned and that cellulite has almost gone.
- Seeing yourself look better can be enough to keep you on the right track.

h. Taking pictures
- You might have seen a number of success stories accompanied with before and after pictures. This is actually a very convenient and effective way to monitor your progress since you don't usually notice little changes. Of course the cheesey grins are not mandatory but do add a comic flavour.
- Stand in front of the mirror (in the bathroom or your bedroom) wearing clothes that reveal your profile. Take a picture using your phone or camera of the front view of the body, the side and the back. You can also take pictures that focus on your problem areas, like your thighs or your stomach.
- You may not want to show these to anyone but try to take pictures every week, or every time you take your numerical measurements. Compile them in your computer with corresponding dates.
- If you go through your weekly pictures, this will give you an idea how your body is changing and if your body is transitioning in accordance to your goals.

- o If you wanted to you could share these on social media so your firned and family can watch your progress, encourage you and keep you accountable to your goals.

i. Clothes fitting
- o Before you start, try to find the clothes that you would want to wear on a regular basis but can't because of your current appearance and health level.
- o As you progress, notice how your body is transitioning and how these clothes fit a little differently weeks ago.

Rewarding Yourself

This is the best part. You need (yes, **need)** to reward yourself in some way, once you reach your specific goals. This will be your source of pleasure; a good experience that would keep you motivated to make more goals and continue your healthy lifestyle.

Aside from the obvious and satisfying rewards of thinking, feeling, and looking better while on the process of reaching your fitness goals, you should also provide yourself with rewards to mark your successes. Try to think hard about what you enjoy doing or things that make you feel good and list them down.

Before you even start working towards your specific goals, try to identify what reward you want to give yourself if you reach it. This would not only improve your focus but will also motivate you all the more. The bigger your goal (which usually are long-term) the grander your reward should be.

Here are some reward suggestions (small and grand) to celebrate your fitness victories:

Do
1. Document your milestones.
   - You can make a scrapbook, photo album or journal every time you reach your goal.
   - For example, when you finally reach your goal weight, snap a picture and file it. You can decorate it and write your positive affirmations.
2. Get a massage or go to a spa to be pampered.
3. Earn an extra hour of sleep.
4. Have a cookout with the whole family.
5. Read and immerse yourself with a good book.
6. Play your favorite game, may it be a board game, computer game or a game done outdoors.
7. Have a long and satisfying bath.
8. Try a different exercise class.
9. Watch your favorite movie or TV series.

10. Take the day off and enjoy a staycation.

Go

1. Go somewhere you always wanted to go to: a restaurant, park, café, etc.
2. Go on a weekend getaway with your friends, loved ones or even alone.
3. Go for a fun hike.
4. Go to a stand-up comedy club or preform a stand up routine.
5. Go to a concert of your favorite band.
6. Go to a movie date with someone or with yourself.
7. Go to a museum or gallery not visited before.
8. Go and watch a sports event that you enjoy.

Chapter 2

The Importance of Good Nutrition

As the saying goes, "It takes two to tango". Your exercise and nutrition go hand in hand. If you're thinking of fad diets that promise that you'll lose fat over a certain span of time (ever heard of 'lose weight in 2 weeks with this diet!'), no, this is not the proper plan that you should follow if you're planning to get strong, fit and healthy. Eating healthily is actually not hard, bland or even restrictive. You just have to eat a balanced diet of good quality protein, carbs and fats. Remember that the type, amount and the quality of the food you eat are used to nourish your body; the better food you take in, the more good it does to your body. A healthy, balanced diet means you'll be receiving enough fuel and nutrients that will make you more energetic, make you look and feel good, make you less at risk from certain diseases and make you live a better quality of life.

The common fad diets of cutting completely out certain food groups i.e. cards are often short-term diets. As with a balanced diet it will be difficult to avoid food groups and possibly need too much will power to stick to them. I have seen friends who have lost a lot of weight on diets like these but of course when they stopped they put the weight straight back on or yo-yoed back and forth with their weight as they started and stopped the dieting. It will be easier to keep a balanced diet that includes the things you like and some treats now again rather than extreme cuts in particular food types.

Food Quality: What You Should Eat

When it comes to the proper diet, the type of food that you eat is of great importance. Which one do you think is better: (two people who consume the same number of calories a day) a person who has consumed sugary doughnuts for breakfast, a burger for lunch and a take-out pizza for dinner or the other who ate whole wheat bread and fruits for breakfast, baked salmon and salad for lunch and lean steak for dinner?

The quality of the food that you eat will also dictate if you'll be fat, sickly and out of shape or lean, healthy and fit.

Your Macronutrients

Our diet is composed of three macronutrients namely proteins, carbohydrates and fat. Fad diets usually eliminate a certain macronutrient group, fat or carb, to facilitate weight loss. However, this is very unhealthy and may take a toll on your longer term health.

You should eat a balanced ratio of protein, carbohydrates and fats. The macronutrient ratio suggestion for a healthy diet is 30:30:40 (30% protein, 30% fat, 40% carbohydrates) if you want to maintain your weight. However, you can manipulate this according to your goals. If you want to bulk up, you can adjust it to say, 30:25:45. If you want to lose weight, you can have the ratio of 40:30:30. These ratios are just suggestions yet these will give you an idea of what to eat more and what to eat less of so that you can stay in line with your goals. Contrary to the common belief that building muscle or losing fat depends solely on the kind of exercise, nutrition plays a much larger role in controlling how you want your body to look.

Carbohydrates

Carbohydrates are the first and easiest source of our body's fuel. Carbohydrates are classified into sugars (simple carbohydrates), and starches (complex carbohydrates). Some familiar carbohydrates include bread, pasta, rice, oats, wheat, barley, cereal, vegetables, fruits, and sweets. Upon intake, these carbohydrate sources are broken down into glucose and is either used for energy or stored.

As there are different kinds of carbohydrates, the rates of their absorption to the bloodstream also differ. The rate of absorption of carbohydrates to the blood is measured by their glycemic index. Carbs that are broken down and absorbed faster, can cause a rapid increase in the release of insulin. This, in turn, will result to your body choosing to store fat and cause spikes and drops in your blood sugar which results to energy crashes and cravings. This is why high glycemic carbohydrates make you hungry after a short period of time, makes you crave more carbohydrates, and eventually leads you to overeat. On the other hand, carbs that are broken down and absorbed slower can stabilize both your blood sugar and insulin levels. You should also consider the nutrient content of the carbohydrates that you eat. When choosing what carb to eat, consider its fiber and nutrients content. Refined and heavily processed carbohydrates (think anything white) get a really bad reputation because they are stripped off of nutrients for aesthetic purposes.

The takeaway: Choose low glycemic, high fiber, nutrient-rich, unrefined, whole carbohydrates. Avoid carbohydrates that have high glycemic index, too much added sugar and are heavily processed and refined.

Eat more of these!
1. Fruits
2. Vegetables
3. Milk
4. Whole grain products: wheat, rye, oats, barley

Eat less of these!
1. Sweetened juices (one option is to have 50/50 water and juice to lower the amount you drink)
2. Any food with refined sugar/corn syrup
3. Sweets
4. Pastries and confectionary

5. Pancakes, muffins, doughnuts, cookies/biscuits
6. Soda/fizzy pop drinks
7. White bread, pasta, cereals

Fat

Dietary fat, in itself, is not the culprit of making people fat. In fact, since the energy in fat is more concentrated, it gives twice the amount of energy given by either carbohydrates or proteins. It is essential in your diet as it improves your overall fitness performance and improves your satisfaction, making you full and satisfied for a longer period of time.

There are actually three types of dietary fat: saturated, unsaturated and trans fats. Saturated fats come from animal and dairy products and all foods with hydrogenated oil (think all fried and fast foods). They are linked to heart diseases because they tend to increase bad cholesterol and triglyceride levels. Trans fats are artificial fats used to extend the shelf life of processed food and foods with shortening/hydrogenated oils (think fast food and baked goods). These kinds of fats are the worse since it lowers your good cholesterol and raises both your bad cholesterol and triglyceride levels, putting you at a high risk of a lot of cardiovascular diseases. On the other hand, unsaturated fats are the healthier ones because they lower your both your bad cholesterol and triglyceride levels. Healthy, unsaturated fat sources include nuts, seeds and fish.

The takeaway: Choose healthy, unsaturated fats. Avoid saturated fat and trans fats.

Eat more of these!
1. Nuts: Peanuts, walnuts, pecans, almonds, etc (use these to replace your sugary snacks)
2. Seeds: flax seeds, chia seeds, sunflower seeds, etc.
3. Oils: olive oil
4. Avocado
5. Fish

Eat less of these!
1. Fast food: french fries, burger, etc
2. Baked goods: cookies, cakes, pastries
3. Processed meat: hotdogs, sausages, bacon, luncheon meats
4. Microwave meals and Junk food

Protein

Protein is the macronutrient made up of amino acids; the building blocks that facilitate the growth and repair of our body's cells: skin, tendons, muscles etc. Amino acids are also important in the synthesis of enzymes, hormones and antibodies and important in the balance of fluids and the regulation of acids and bases. Protein is basically essential everywhere in our body.

Lean and healthy proteins are the stars of the diets of healthy and fit people. This is because they facilitate repair, improve satiety, and adequate intake enables your body to maintain and build your muscles. Upon eating protein, you also feel full fast, which in turn, makes you eat less overall. Healthy protein choices include lean meats, fish, eggs, beans and tofu.

When you are trying to maintain or build muscle, ideally, you have to consume 1-1.5 grams of protein per pound weight. For example, if you are a lightly active adult woman, who aims to build muscle and weighs 125 pounds, you should eat about 125 grams of protein a day.

The takeaway: Eat enough protein daily and get them from lean and low-fat sources.

Eat More of These!
1. Lean Meats: Pork, Lamb, beef, etc (leanest and protein-rich part: parts of loin or round)
2. Poultry: chicken or turkey (leanest and protein-rich part: breast)
3. Legumes: beans, peas and lentils
4. Eggs
5. Dairy products: Milk, cheese, yogurt

Eat Less of These!
1. Processed and fatty meat
2. High sugar dairy products
3. Fatty cuts of meat

Food Quantity: How Much You Should Eat

Apart from the type of food that you eat, how much you eat is equally important. Even though you eat healthy foods, if you consume a lot (say, 5 eggs and a whole pack of whole wheat bread for a meal) you'll still gain weight.

Although I don't count calories below is an example of how to do this if you want to. For me I just want the ease of simple measurements I can use to cook quickly with and not have to measure every single item. The more complicated cooking becomes the more likley you are to become frustrated, demotivated and revert to poor habits. Further on we will look at some of the quick ways to measure out food quickly.

Calories

Calories are the amount of energy that our body obtains from the food we eat. Your body needs a certain number of calories per day to function. If you consume above your recommended intake, the excess calories will be stored. If you consume less, the deficit will help you lose the excess fat.

So, then how much calories do you need each day? To be able to know how much you should eat for your day to day bodily functions, you need to calculate the number of calories you should consume.

Your total caloric requirement involves two major factors: your basal metabolic rate (BMR) and your physical activity levels (PAL).

As a general rule of thumb, you can roughly estimate your daily caloric requirement (at resting state or your Basal Metabolic Rate) by multiplying your weight (in pounds) by 12 for males or 11 for females. Understand that this is only a rough approximation and many factors can affect your recommended daily calorie intake. However, this will give you an idea of how much you should eat.

For example:

Caloric requirement 155 pound man = 155 pounds x 12 = 1,860 calories/day (BMR)

Caloric requirement 125 pound woman = 125 pounds x 11 = 1,375 calories/day (BMR)

The above estimation is only for the calories that you need for your body to function properly; just enough fuel for essential bodily processes such as breathing, digestion, processes in the brain, etc. When estimating how many calories you need a day, you also have to consider your physical activity levels (PAL). Your PAL is a number that you multiply with your BMR.

Here is a guideline of your factor-translated physical activity levels:

1. Sedentary (not much activity, sitting all day): 1.2
2. Lightly active (light exercise once or twice a week): 1.3
3. Moderately active (moderate exercise twice or thrice a week): 1.4
4. Active (moderate exercise more than thrice a week): 1.6
5. Vigorously active (intense exercise six to seven times a week): 1.7

Now that you know how to estimate how many calories your body needs to function optimally and how many it needs for your physical activity, you can now estimate your total caloric requirement.

Total caloric requirement = Caloric requirement (BMR) x Physical Activity Level (PAL)

In theory, a moderately active person should consume 2,000-2,800 calories to sustain all essential body processes and physical activity.

The 'calorie in, calorie out' premise indicates that to maintain your weight, the amount of calories that you take in should be equal to the amount that your body uses to function plus the amount you expend in physical activity.

To **maintain your weight**, your calorie intake should be equal to your calorie expenditure:

Calorie intake = Calorie expenditure (bodily functions + physical activity)

To **gain weight**, your calorie intake should be more than your calorie expenditure. Theoretically, you should increase your total calorie intake by 20% to gain weight.

Calorie intake > Calorie expenditure (bodily functions + physical activity)

To **lose weight**, your calorie intake should be less than your calorie expenditure.

Theoretically, you should decrease your total calorie intake by 15% to lose weight. *Calorie intake < Calorie expenditure (bodily functions + physical activity)*

Portions and Serving Sizes

Even though you already know how many calories you should eat, as mentioned before some people (incldung myself) still view calorie counting as tedious work. In fact, some may feel that they are restricting themselves too much, especially those whose goal is to lose weight.

Another alternative to calorie counting is estimating the portions of your food. Though less accurate than counting calories, estimating portions can help you regulate the amount of your food intake, in relation to your daily requirement.

Estimating Serving Sizes and Portions

Serving sizes often come in the measurements like tablespoons, cups (often more of an American serving), ounces, grams, etc. It is the suggested, standard amount of food that you eat. A portion, on the other hand, is the amount of food you choose to eat.

When it comes to controlling the amount of food that you eat, you have to estimate how many calories that food contains by comparing it to familiar items. If you aim to lose weight, estimating portions can be very useful since you need to eat less than your recommended intake and or probably less than you used to eat, or less of what you used to eat i.e. fatty sugary foods.

Use this guide to estimate your portions:

1. Closed fist/ tennis ball
   - 1 cup
   - A serving of rice, pasta, fruit or vegetable
   - 1/3 serving of air-popped popcorn
2. Light bulb
   - ½ cup
   - Half a serving of cooked rice or pasta
3. Whole palm/ deck of cards
   - 3 ounces
   - An adequate serving of protein
   - A serving of meat, fish, or poultry
4. Thumb
   - 1 ounce
   - A serving of peanut butter or cheese
5. Tip of your thumb
   - 1 teaspoon
   - A serving of cooking oil, mayonnaise or butter
6. Handful

- 1 ounce, ½ cup
- A serving of nuts or raisins
- Half a cup of cooked beans
7. Two Handfuls
   - A serving/ 1 cup of vegetable salad
8. Flat hand
   - One serving/one slice of bread

Of course the above is just a rough guide and should/could be adapted compared to your needs and goals. It does however give a quicker way to measure food portions.

Nutrition Labels
Looking at nutrition labels is another useful practice that could aid you in controlling the amount and kind of food that you eat. Whenever you buy groceries, notice the small table at the back or sometimes front of pre-packed goods. This is called the Nutrition Label or the Nutrition Facts. This list contains the total calories of the item (or the total calories in a serving), the number of grams of each macronutrient (Total Fat, Total Carbs, Protein) contained in the item, and the additional components such as sugar, saturated fat, trans fat, sodium, fiber, iron, Vitamin C, etc. Check the total amount of calories per serving, the macronutrients and the nutritional content of your food. Limit foods high in saturated fat, trans fat and sugar. Now adays they are also helpfully colour coded with red or orange indicating high levels f one thing or another. Obviously if its high in salt/suger/fat you can review if there might be healthier options.
Tips for Estimating and Limiting Portions
1. Read nutrition labels.
2. Eat slowly and mindfully.

   As you put the food into your mouth, savor and chew it well.

   When you appreciate your food, you tend to eat slower and you'll easily notice if you're already full. This way, you can avoid overeating.

3. Use smaller plates.

   The bigger the plate the more you eat, and smaller plates trick the mind to thinking that you're already eating a lot when in fact you're eating the right portions. Its very common if not ingrained in you as a child to eat everything on your plate. So the more you pile on your plate the more likley you are to try and eat it all.

4. Drink a glass of water before you eat.

   This makes you feel fuller before you start mindlessly chugging down that burger.

5. Serve appropriate serving sizes when cooking at home.

Have serving cups ready at home for proper serving sizes.

6. Avoid distractions while eating

    Focus on what and how much you're eating.

    Avoid distractions such as television, phones and other electronic gadgets which can aid in mindless eating.

7. Split your order when dining out.

    Serving sizes in restaurants are ridiculously large and are usually two to three times more than you should eat.

    Split a large meal with your friend, or if you're eating alone, request the half as a take-out and eat it for another meal.

12. You can slow your ordering in the sense that you order one course at a time to guage your hunger rather than ordering all 3 courses at once and then ploughing your way through them regardless of being full or not.

8. Eat your vegetables first.

    Try to eat your veggies first to make you feel full at the start of the meal.

    And if you are like me and don't like vegetables it gets them over and done with at the beginning and ensures you eat them rather than pushing them around the plate till you give up.

Meal Timing: When You Should Eat

At different times of the day, our bodies have different metabolic needs. In your diet and fitness journey, it is important to properly nourish your body with the right nutrients that it needs at certain times of the day. Meal timing is based on this premise and it suggests the kind of food that you should eat at different times of the day to maximize fat loss and fitness or muscle building.

Morning: Breakfast

Body's State: After hours of sleep, your body is in a fasted state. This means that your carb energy stores are low, your muscles are in the midst of wasting, and your fat stores are slowly being burned by the body.

Goals of Breakfast: To compensate, your morning nutrition should resupply your carbohydrate stores, stop possible muscle wasting, and encourage the further burning of your fat stores.

Breakfast Nutrition: Your breakfast should consist protein, carbohydrates and fat. Consume high quality and easily absorbed protein, like eggs, to provide amino acids to the almost wasting muscles. To replenish your carbohydrate stores, eat a mix of simple and complex carbohydrates, like fruits and whole grains. Lastly, a small part of your meal should contain healthy fats from nuts, or seeds like flax and chia.

You will also likley be fairly dehydrated, so a glass of water or 50/50 fruit juice and water would be a good start to rehydrating.

Morning: Snack

Body's State: At mid-morning, your body has already used up half of your replenished carbohydrate stores so your blood sugar is already getting low and you'd start to feel hungry.

Goals of Morning Snack: Your nutrition by this time should support the maintenance of your muscles and stabilize your blood sugar levels.

Morning Snack Nutrition: You should eat a snack of mixed protein source, like milk, and eat a low glycemic index carbohydrate to maintain the levels of your blood sugar. Or in plain English, fresh fruits or vegetables, dried fruits and or nuts.

Lunch

Body's State: At midday, your body has already adjusted and is probably in a balanced state already.

Goals of Lunch: The goal is just to maintain this balanced state, continue the support for the muscles and maintain a stabilized blood sugar level.

Lunch Nutrition: Your lunch should again contain a good balance of protein, carbohydrates and essential fats. Choose lean protein sources like poultry, fish or meat to provide your muscles with fast-acting amino-acids. Unlike breakfast, eat your lunch with low glycemic index carbohydrates like whole grains. Also, make sure you get a dose of essential fatty acids in the form of healthy fats. One good example is a small serving of cottage cheese.

Afternoon: Snack

Body's State: During the afternoon, your blood sugar levels are probably running low and your muscles are again on the verge of wasting.

Goals of Afternoon Snack: Your afternoon snack should bring your blood sugar at a stable level and provide a good amount of amino acids for your muscles.

Afternoon Snack Nutrition: Eat a small snack that contains slow-acting protein and with carbohydrate component that's low on sugar but has a medium glycemic index. An unsweetened nutrition bar can do the trick.

Night: Dinner

Body's State: Dinner is the last meal of the day and it will be your body's source of nutrition during your hours of sleep. Overnight, your muscles will first undergo healing, or muscle-building for the first couple of hours. However, in the succeeding hours, your body will start using up your energy stores: carb, fat and protein.

Goals of Dinner: Your dinner should be able to provide nutrition to support muscle building and prevent muscle wasting all throughout the night. It should also shift your body's focus to burning fat and carb stores instead of your protein stores.

Dinner Nutrition: Eat slow-acting proteins that will provide your muscles ample supply of amino acids while you sleep. This includes high quality protein like lean meat, poultry, beef, lamb or pork. The carbohydrate part of your meal should be high in fiber and of low glycemic index, like a serve of salad greens. Have another dose of healthy fats, too. You can opt to drizzle your salad with an appropriate serving of olive oil.

Pre-workout Snack

Body's State: Before your workout, your body is in need of ample energy source to sustain your physical activity.

Goals of Pre-workout Snack: The main objective of your pre-workout snack should be to provide a fuel source throughout your workout. It should also maintain your energy levels and prevent the wasting of your muscles.

Pre-workout Snack Nutrition: Eaten 30 minutes to an hour before the workout, your pre-workout snack should be composed of complex and high-fiber carbohydrates and an appropriate amount of fast-acting proteins. You can have a slice of whole wheat bread with a poached egg, or a banana topped with a nut butter.

Post-workout Snack

Body's State: After working out, your muscles has already undergone a certain amount of degradation.

Goals of Post-workout Snack: Your post-workout snack nutrition should replenish your protein sources and repair your muscles. It should also replace the fluids lost in the activity.

Post-workout Snack Nutrition: Eat a snack with protein and carbohydrates (mix of simple and complex). Avoid foods high and fat and if possible, eat less of fibrous carbohydrates. A good post-workout meal can be turkey breast with sweet potatoes.

Easy take aways

- Carry healthy snacks with you so you don't get caught out and head for the chocolate
- Substitute chocolates and biscuits – especially in the office environment where you can easy chomp through snacks while just sitting at your desk
- Easily measure out your portions and keep to eating enough and not all you can.
- Eating from smaller plates or only filling a part of the plate can help control portion sizes.

Water Wonders

Hydration is probably one of the most important things in health and fitness but unfortunately, also one of the most neglected areas. Naturally through the day you need to hydrate, important times can be after a nights sleep, ongoing during the day, with meals and especially when you work out.

Im actually not a big water drinker and often have to force myself at times to drink more. But without fail the longer I go without drinking water the more likley I am to feel tired, lethargic and eventually to end up with a headache. Therefore I have now taken to drinking a large glass of water when I wake up, with every meal and every other time I have a drink of tea/cofee. This way through habit I have begun to drink more water. The only caveat have is that I try not to drink to much water just before bed for obvious reasons. As my father used to say a cup of water at night leads to a cup of wee wee at night.

When you work out, your body heats up and to get rid of the excess heat, you sweat and lose body fluids. This will then lead to dehydration which can cause fatigue in muscles, decrease performance in fitness routines and loss of coordination.

You should make sure that you are drinking enough water all throughout the day, especially before, during and after your workouts. Ideally, you should drink about 6-8 glasses or at least 2 liters of water a day. However, if you are working out, you should be drinking more as you lose more fluids and salts throughout the physical activity.

Around 15 minutes before your workout, drink 250-350 ml of water to sustain your hydration needs during the exercise. You can also add a pinch of salt to help replenish the salts that you lose together with the fluids.

During the exercise, drink around 80-100 ml every thirty minutes of activity. Make sure that you don't drink more than a liter per hour as this can lead to over-hydration.

Within two hours after your exercise, drink about 500-100mL of water to replenish the fluids that your body lost.

To know if you are properly hydrated, you should not rely on your thirst. You should check the color of your urine. The darker your urine the more dehydrated you are. If your urine is of pale yellow color, you are properly hydrated.

Rest/Recovery Days

Why you need to take a rest from your workouts

Resting might sound counterproductive, but your rest days are just as important as your workout itself. This is because your muscles are damaged during workouts and your body needs time to heal and regenerate them, to build them and make them stronger.

What to eat on rest days

A rest day is not a cheat day. You should give your body proper nutrition to support the processes that are happening when you're not working out. The quality and the quantity of your nutrition on rest days should support muscle building and nutrient replenishment and encourage further fat loss.

Caloric cycling is a technique wherein your nutrition is different during rest and work out days to address the body's specific needs based on your activity per day. Generally, you should eat slightly less than your recommended caloric intake on rest days to encourage fat loss and eat more protein to maximize muscle building. On your workout days, eat just enough calories to sustain your body's functional needs and your physical activity. You should also focus on eating the proper ratio of protein and carbohydrates to fuel your body up and avoid muscle wasting.

On your rest day, aim to eat protein on all your three big meals. Focus on lean and healthy protein sources like fish, eggs, and poultry. These should give you ample amount of amino acids to help rebuild your muscles. Also, aim to eat a complex carbohydrate on only one meal of the day and load your plate up with vegetables for all three meals.

What to do on rest days

How often you should rest and what you should do during this time is dictated by the intensity of your workouts for the whole week. If you are exercising moderately 3-4 days a week, you should not have complete rest periods where you don't do anything active. Instead, have active recovery days doing low-intensity and low-impact physical activities that complement the bodyweight exercises you did all throughout the week.

Focus on cardio and flexibility on your rest days. You can do light aerobic activities like Zumba, light jogging, or even long walks just to keep your heart pumping and improve circulation. You can also take the chance to improve your flexibility and balance during your rest days. Yoga is one of the most ideal exercises to do on your days off since it stretches and lengthens your muscles and tendons. This soothes the sore and tightened up muscles that you get from working out and also improves your recovery, flexibility and mobility overall.

However, if you do high-intensity and heavy training for 6 days a week, you can probably take a complete rest day. You shouldn't be completely sedentary, though. You can take a short walk in the park, a yoga session or have a massage to soothe those sore muscles.

Most importantly, have fun during your rest days! Find something active to do alone or with your friends or family. You can go on camping, hiking or even go for a little swim. As long as you don't stay sedentary, your imagination is the limit for things to do off of your workout schedule.

Chapter 3

Fitness and Bodyweight Workout Basics

Health: A Fitness Aspect

What does it mean to be healthy and fit? Is it all about your weight, height or physical appearance?

Being fit is more than that. Health-related physical fitness is known to be the overall state wherein your body can easily perform certain bodily tasks. Generally, it is composed of five main components: cardiovascular endurance, muscular strength, muscular endurance, body composition, and flexibility. In addition to these, balance and coordination are also of important consideration.

1. **Cardiovascular endurance**: your ability to do any activity that increases the heart rate for a period of time, usually for at least twenty minutes or more
2. **Muscular strength**: the ability of your muscles to exert maximum force against a weight or a resistance
3. **Muscular endurance**: the ability of your muscles to perform a certain range of motion repeatedly without getting exhausted
4. **Body composition**: the ratio of your lean muscle mass to your body fat
5. **Flexibility**: your ability to bend and move with your joints through a full range of motion
6. **Balance:** your ability to maintain your body's central gravity and stay in control of body movement
7. **Coordination:** your ability to combine a number of actions in a single movement

Exercise is one of the main factors that can improve your physical health. There are quite a number of types of exercises and the broadest of them includes cardiovascular exercises, lifting weights and as we will go on to talk about bodyweight workouts. These workout classifications include thousands of exercises that target different areas of your physical health. Though it is true that there is no "perfect workout" that applies to everyone, finding out which one fits you best and which one you can stick with, will do wonders to your health and well-being.

What are Bodyweight Workouts?

Consistency or forming good habits are the most important factors if your goal is to become and stay fit. Workouts shouldn't be too much of a hassle so that it becomes a chore, a few small lifestyle changes can help you reap all the health benefits of being more active and forming positive mental and physical fitness habits

So, is there a fitness regimen that's easy to stick to, convenient, can be performed anywhere and anytime, and most of all, free? The answer is a resounding **YES!** It is in the form of bodyweight workouts.

Bodyweight workouts, as suggested by its name, are exercises that make use of your own body weight as a form of resistance. Almost like weightlifting, bodyweight workouts work on exerting a substantial amount of force on a weight, in this case your own, to shed excess fat and build your muscles.

Nowadays, though the trend of getting fit is widespread and even 'contagious', although it often ends up with people spending too much on expensive gym equipment, gym memberships and fad diets that never last. One of the most effective ways to lose fat and build lean muscle is often overlooked: forming positive nutrition habits and using our own body to exercise.

Bodyweight workouts are generally ideal for people who are interested in improving their overall fitness; that is improving cardiovascular endurance, muscle strength and endurance, flexibility, balance, coordination and body composition. Through these routines, endurance can be improved by increasing the number of repetitions, strength can be improved by increasing the intensity or the difficulty of execution, and flexibility and body composition can be improved through full-range of motion exercises.

Bodyweight Workouts vs. Cardio Exercises

Cardiovascular exercises are usually done to improve your heart's endurance. They are a set of workouts that involve any kind of activity that increases your heart rate over an extended period of time. Some of the most basic cardio exercises include jogging, running, swimming and cycling.

Cardio exercises are deemed to be the most effective way to lose fat. This is because the body uses your carbohydrate sources first as fuel and after all these are depleted, it switches to burning the body's fat stores. However, after continuous cardiovascular exertion, protein is the next in line to be used. Prolonged exercise through these steady-state cardio workouts can lead to muscle loss. This is why marathoners are usually thin. In fact, some of those who lost weight only from cardio have saggy and lose skin. You wouldn't want your exercises only targeting the cardiovascular system; it should also involve all the other components of health-related fitness.

In bodyweight exercises, you can both lose fat and maintain and even build your muscles. Unlike cardio exercises, bodyweight exercises can trigger the release of hormones that speed up your metabolic rate: growth hormone and testosterone. A high metabolic rate makes you effectively lose fat, because you continuously burn calories, even 48 hours after your last workout, making your routine very efficient. Also, as you are improving your muscles' endurance and strength by subjecting your body to the resistance that is your own weight, muscle wasting is prevented.

The traditional cardiovascular exercises undertaken include running, tread mills, step machines etc. Depending on your interest in running, age, existing fitness and or injuries this may or may not be a good place to start. Like myself I have seen many people determined to lose weight or get fit start running often in gym equipment not having seen the light of day since they left school or university. It's often nothing but a painful and self-defeating exercise unless you have some burning motivation i.e charity half or full marathon to aim for driving you on. Of course running can form part of your exercise routine but for me it is and has only been a part and often small.

Walking to fitness

An easier gentler start is to start walking!! What? But I already do they everyday I hear you say! Well yes most if not everyone walks everyday but not many of us do enough of it to have any beneficial effects. For it to have any health benefits you have to feel like you have done some walking and done some exercise

There is much debate about how much walking is the minimum or best amount for any actual health benefits but generally its seems to have settled more or less around 10,000 steps. This is approximately 7km, of course this depends on your stride length but is a rough ball park figure. At this level you would start to notice the walking i.e. it would likely require you to consciously go for a walk. If you work in an office largely sat down all day you would need to go for a walk at breaks and lunches.

For me I though walking would be a good way to start getting fit, didn't require any equipment other than the shoes I already had and could be done easily everyday.

I originally started with a target of 8000 steps per day. At the beginning I had no idea how far 8000 steps would be, I thought that must be far, its in the thousands. For my daily commute I have to walk to the station and then at the other side to my office and often go for a walk in my lunch hour to get some fresh air, British weather permitting. I also took the opportunity to walk up any steps I needed to avoid the lift and walked to people's desks instead of emailing or calling them. With this I found that 8000 steps was easily achievable so I upped it to 10000.

With 10000 steps I began to find that I needed to consciously undertake my normal walking but also look for additional walking opportunities in lunches and breaks. My slight cheat is that I now try and walk an average of 10000 steps per day per week; with my walking app this is easy to track.

Of course its difficult to attribute was it the diet, additional exercise or the walking that has helped me to start losing weight and feeling fitter, most likely it's a combination of them all over time.

So give it a go, get a walking app, step counter and start your walking exercises.

Walking cheats

- Look for opportunities to walk all the time i.e. walk up the steps and dont take lifts or escalators or at least walk up the escalators.
- Walk to the shops – even if they are further away maybe use the time to listen to podcasts or music
- Resolve to do your shopping on foot and walk as much of it as possible
- Take a walk during breaks and lunches – you can use this time to explore new areas of plan the rest of your day.

- If friends come round suggesting walking and talking.
- You can easily purchase an inexpensive step counter or download the many free walking apps on your smart phone.

Bodyweight Workouts vs. Weight Lifting

One common myth when doing bodyweight workouts is that you can't make a lot of progress when compared to lifting weights at the gym. First things first, though, how is bodyweight training different from weight training?

In the simplest sense, the principle of both training regimens is the same: you make your muscles exert force against a resistance, in both cases, a weight. When you subject your muscles to a resistance, it is worn out and eventually damaged. When the body naturally heals them, it comes back stronger to be able to adapt to stress.

In weight lifting, you usually need equipment (dumbbells, barbells, etc) and/or machines. As your muscles adapt to the weight that you're lifting, you need to move to a heavier weight to make sure that you are making progress. This process is called progressive overloading wherein you increase the weight to increase the stress to your muscles. Adding weight to increase the intensity of your workout would lead to muscle strength gains and muscle enlargement.

Progressive overload is seen as one of the advantage of weight training over bodyweight workouts, since you can just increase your weights to ensure progress. However, the thing is, your body doesn't discriminate the type of weight that you subject your muscles to. Whether its barbells or your own weight, the effect will still be same as long as it's the same amount of load. Also, by performing difficult versions of bodyweight exercises, progressive overload is possible. If you're a beginner in strength training or you just do not have access to weights, doing bodyweight exercises is a good way to go.

One advantage of bodyweight exercises over weight lifting is that it doesn't subject the body to external stress; you're just using your own weight. Since our bodies are not designed to endure very heavy loads, weightlifters usually develop joint problems over time. Bodyweight training also focuses on improving other components of fitness such as agility, coordination and flexibility. These components are not easily improved by weight training of isolated muscles wherein only a certain part of the body is subjected to a resistance. Training using your body weight usually involves compound movements or movements that involve different parts of your body at the same time, improving your overall fitness.

Benefits of Bodyweight Workouts

Do it anytime, anywhere

- When it comes to getting fit, no one has time for complication. In fitness, the key to success is convenience so that you can make sure that you won't fall prey to your excuses. Your schedules shouldn't be a large hindrance to your fitness regimen.

- Using little to no equipment, bodyweight exercises can be done anytime and anywhere you want. Every exercise using your own body can be adjusted to adapt to whatever situation you are in.
    o Travelling or on a business trip? You can do pushups and squats in your hotel room.
    o Crunched for time? Do 10 burpees tor star jumps to keep your heart pumping and feel the burn in your muscles.
    o Don't want to leave the house? There are hundreds of efficient exercises to try at home.
    o No access to weights or the gym? Your body is your gym. Creativity can go a long way since you can use simple household items to spice up your workouts.
    o Sat on the coach in between adverts – drop down and do 5,10 press ups before the programme restarts.
    o No need to pack kit bags or spend time travelling to the gym.
- With bodyweight exercises, you only need a small space, a little time and a little bit of determination.

No to excuses! Yes to consistency!

- Convenience is next to consistency. When you're doing something that doesn't require a lot of hassle and complication, it's more likely that you'll do it regularly!
- Remember, the journey to being fit and healthy is not a speed race, but a marathon. It should be a part of your routine and your lifestyle.
- Excuses such as not having enough time, being too tired, or not having the equipment to use can be easily shrugged off. You have the liberty to choose what time, where and how you do your workouts.

Absolutely Free!

- Who said being fit and healthy needs to be expensive? Even if you have no gym membership, no heavy or expensive equipment or weights, and no branded gym clothes, you can still reap the benefits of exercising using bodyweight workouts.

- All you need is something that you can never go without, your own body!

Strength and Cardio Training: Combined!

- Probably one of the advantages of bodyweight exercises over weight lifting and cardio training is the possibility of combining both.
- You'll hit two birds with one stone: you can have heart blasting exercises while still improving the strength and endurance of your muscles. High-intensity interval training is one example of this perfect workout combination.

Lose fat and build muscle

- Since you can combine both cardio and strength training, it's possible to lose fat and build muscle with bodyweight workouts.
- One common myth in fitness is that you can't lose fat and build muscle at the same time. However, this is highly possible when you have the proper approach to nutrition and efficiently mix cardio and strength in your bodyweight exercises.

Everyone can do it

- Whatever your fitness level, age or body composition, there's a bodyweight exercise routine that's just for you.
- Bodyweight workouts' intensity and level of difficulty are easily customizable to be suitable for your fitness goals and level. There are easier and harder versions of hundreds of these exercises!

Home workouts rock!

- Bodyweight workouts enable you to exercise in the comforts of your home.
- You can avoid embarrassing/skimpy gym outfits and the feeling of people secretly judging you.
- You can work out whenever and wherever you are: in the living room, in the bedroom, in the garden and even in the kitchen! Nothing beats the privacy and the convenience of working out at home.

Improve overall fitness

- Usually, weight trainings and cardio exercises done in the gym only focus one of these three: muscle strength, endurance or cardio endurance.
- In bodyweight workouts, aside from improving the first three, your overall fitness level is also improved.
- In fact, gymnasts train using only their bodyweight and the holistic effect to their athleticism can be seen in their physique and their performance.

   a. Balance
   o To increase the intensity of your workouts, you might need to try more challenging variations of basic bodyweight exercises.
   o These variations often improve balance because they require you to work more on your weight.
   b. Coordination
   o Bodyweight workouts usually employ different parts of the body and different actions in one movement. Doing and practicing them can improve how your whole body work together.
   c. Flexibility
   o Full range of motion movements improves is your flexibility.
   o Increasing the intensity of your workout means doing more challenging positions. This in turn, improves your ability to move and stretch with ease.

Reduced chance of joint injuries

- Since your body is not subjected to heavy and unnatural weights in bodyweight workouts, you decrease your risk of having joint injuries.
- Some heavy weightlifters tend to develop certain joint problems through time because of overexertion and wearing out of joints due to friction. When you come to think of it, lifting too heavy weights has little functionality in our everyday lives. Where as being able to mange your own body weight has daily applicability.

No to monotony

- When you're doing gym workouts, there are times when you become bored. In doing exercises on treadmills or machine equipment, there isn't too much variation that you can do.
- With bodyweight exercises, you wouldn't need to rely on repetitive and somewhat boring programs. You can mix and match different variations, vary the intensity, volume and the lengths in between. You can vary when and where you do it also, at home, in the park, when on holiday in fact anywhere.

Chapter 4

Warming Up and Cooling Down

Before we start with the workouts themselves, it is important to know that your body needs preparation before the workout and toning down after the exercise. More often than not, people neglect the importance of warming up and cooling down, leading to increased risk to injuries and unwanted pain. If you haven't worked out or done fitness training for a long time a proper warn up is crucial for the short term to ensure you don't feel to much stiffness or discomfort after your first session and for the long-term so you don't give up when you feel sore.

Importance of Warming Up

Before a workout, the body needs to be properly warmed up to prep it up for increasing demands of the following physical activity. It prepares the body and the mind for exercises, thus, lessening the chance of both muscle and joint injury. Benefits, warm-up exercises:

- Improves your circulation throughout your body, facilitating the loosening up and the proper oxygenation of your muscles
- Heats the body up and further making the muscles more flexible
- Improves coordination and brain function
- Increase the supply of synovial fluids to the joints to avoid joint injury

Warm-up Exercises

Your warm-up exercises before a bodyweight workout should moderately elevate your heart rate. It should cause you to sweat a little but it shouldn't tire you out. Ideal warm up exercises should heat up your body, reduce muscle stiffness, and improve the pliability of the specific muscles to be used in your workout.

Dynamic Warm Up

Dynamic warm ups require the movement of the whole body and all the joints until the body heats up considerably and the muscles loosen. You would do stretches while moving. These kinds of warm up exercises are perfect for bodyweight training.

Here are some sample exercises that you may want to try. Feel free to adjust the level of difficulty if it feels too easy or too hard.

- Jumping jacks/star jumps for 1 minute
- High knees for 30 seconds
- Arm circles for 30 seconds
- Toe touches for 30 seconds
- Light jog in place for 3 minutes

Importance of Cooling Down

After working out, your body's processes are still at their heights: your heart rate is faster than normal, your breathing is unsteady, your muscles are stiff and contracted and your body temperature is high. Cooling down will help your body return to a normal state at a gradual rate.
Benefits: cool down routine:

- Prevent the pooling of blood in your muscles
- Normalize your heart rate bit by bit
- Ensures proper blood circulation by bringing blood back to the heart and the brain
- Reduce the levels of lactic acid in the blood, preventing excessive muscle soreness

Cooling Down Routines

To aid your body to gradually return to the normal state, cool down by lowering your heart rate first then stretch to reduce the stiffness in your muscles. Stretch your muscles up until you feel a slight discomfort but be careful not to strain. Hold the stretch for about 20-30 seconds.
Heart Rate Lowering

- Walk in place for 5 minutes; or
- Do a light jog while slowly reducing speed

Stretching

- Buttock stretch: Lie down. Bring your knees up to your chest and put your right leg over your left thigh. Grasp the back of your left thigh and pull your right knee to your chest. Repeat for the other leg.
- Toe grab: Sit up and put your toes together so that your legs form a diamond.
- Cobra pose: This yoga pose stretches your back and your core. Lie on your stomach and put both hands in line with your shoulders. Gently and slowly lift yourself up until you feel the stretch.
- Hand down spine: Bring your right hand down the center of your back, your left hand assisting with the stretch. Lean into the stretch. Repeat for the other hand.
- Arm overhead stretch: Interlock your fingers and bring them over your head with palms facing upward.

Chapter 5

Getting fit through Bodyweight Workouts

This chapter contains many of the common bodyweight exercises: how they are executed and how to make them harder or easier. There are pictures of the exercises at the end of this book and you can also do a simple YouTube search will also give you a worked description of all the workouts. Seeing them done will help you improve your form and avoid injury.

You can choose the workouts for a general all over body workout or use them to concentrate on particular areas of the body.

Tips before Starting

1. **Terminologies**
   Repetitions or reps: one movement of an exercise
   Set: consists of the complete number of repetitions (For example: 3 x 12 is 12 repetitions of an exercise to be repeated three times)
   Rest: the amount of time between sets
   Failure: the point wherein you can no longer perform another repetition
   High Intensity Interval Training (HIIT): one of the most effective ways to burn fat and build muscle through bodyweight exercises. It is composed of a cycle of bursts of movement and a period of rest.

2. **Proper Execution**
   Each exercise should be done with proper technique and form. Doing an exercise incorrectly can lead to injury.

3. **Quality over Quantity**
   When doing an exercise, the quality of the exercise is more important than completing the number of repetitions.
   If you feel that you're reaching failure, rest for a few seconds and resume.

4. **Increasing Intensity**
   To increase intensity of your workouts:
   a. Hold fully extended or contracted position as long as you can
   b. Prolong your last rep of the movement. Go as slow as you can, feeling the resistance of your weight.
   c. Pause for three seconds at the most difficult part of the movement.
   d. Do additional reps.
   e. Try a more difficult variation.

5. **Proper breathing**

Inhale during the easy part and exhale during the harder part of the exercise

6. **Convenient equipment around the house**

    Tables, chairs, stairs, boxes, steps: can be used as stable surfaces

    Door/door frames or lying under tables: can be used for pull-ups

    Heavy objects such as books, milk jugs, and bags: can be used as free weights.

Bodyweight Workouts

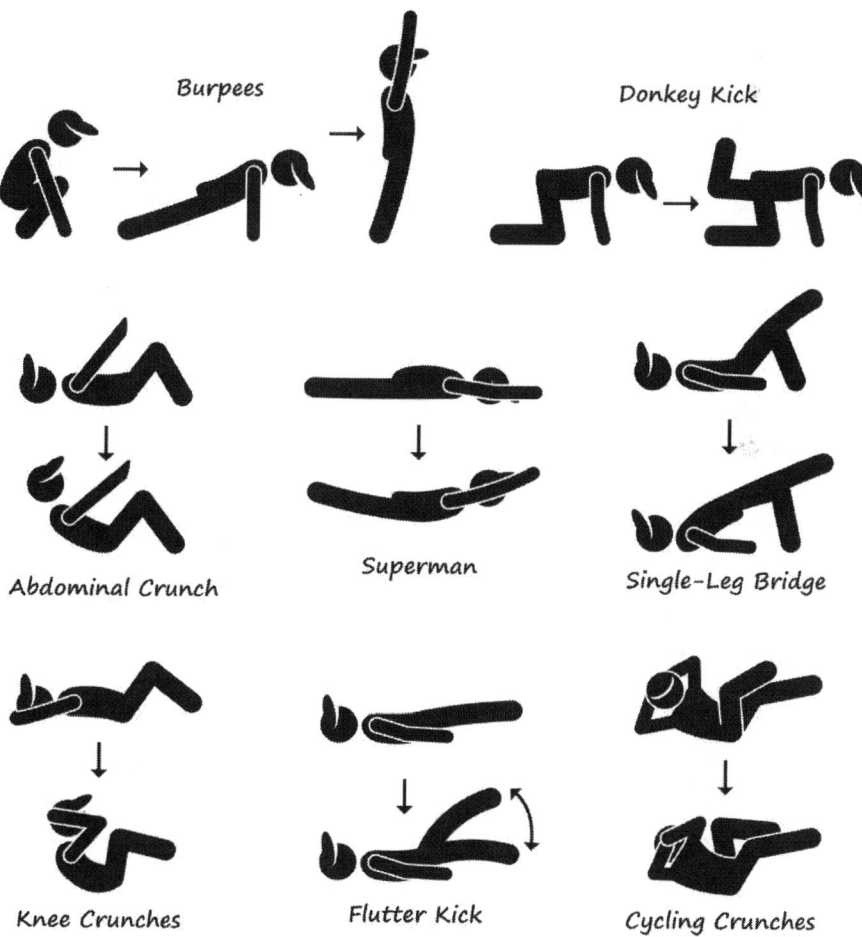

Burpees

Donkey Kick

Abdominal Crunch

Superman

Single-Leg Bridge

Knee Crunches

Flutter Kick

Cycling Crunches

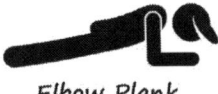

Elbow Plank

Basic Plank

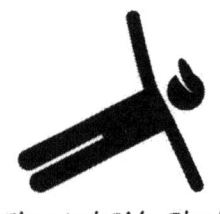

Elevated Side Plank

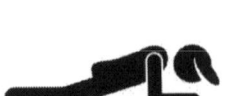

Elbow Plank (Knee)

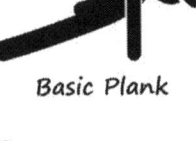

Plank Leg Raise

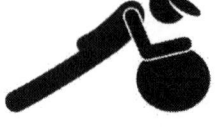

Ball Plank

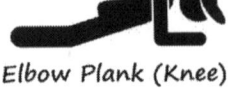

Bent Knee Side Plank

Plank Arm Reach

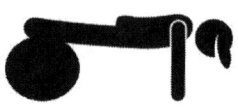

Ball Plank Reverse

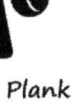

Side Plank

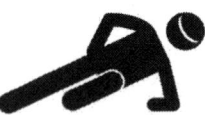

Side Plank
Knee Tuck (1)

Extended Plank

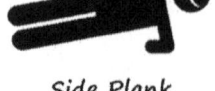

Side Plank Leg Lift

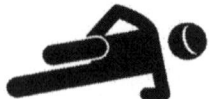

Side Plank
Knee Tuck (2)

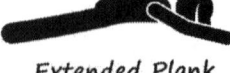

Reverse Plank

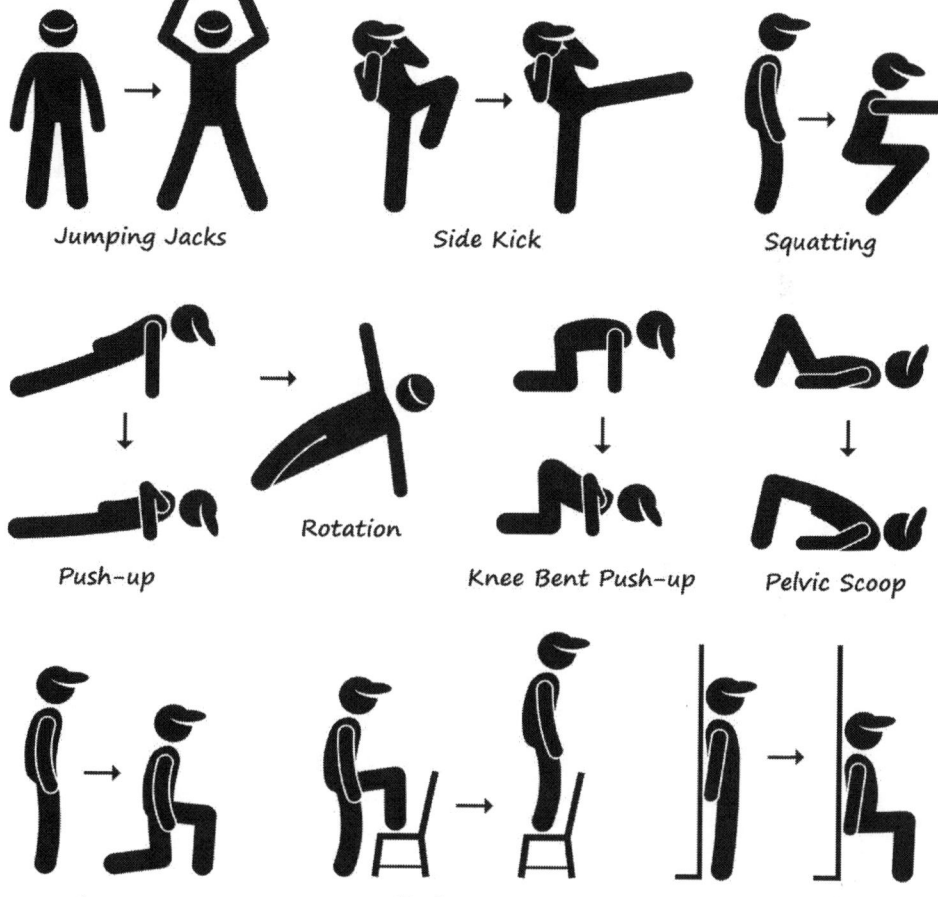

Jumping Jacks

Side Kick

Squatting

Push-up

Rotation

Knee Bent Push-up

Pelvic Scoop

Lunge

Chair Step Up

Wall Sit

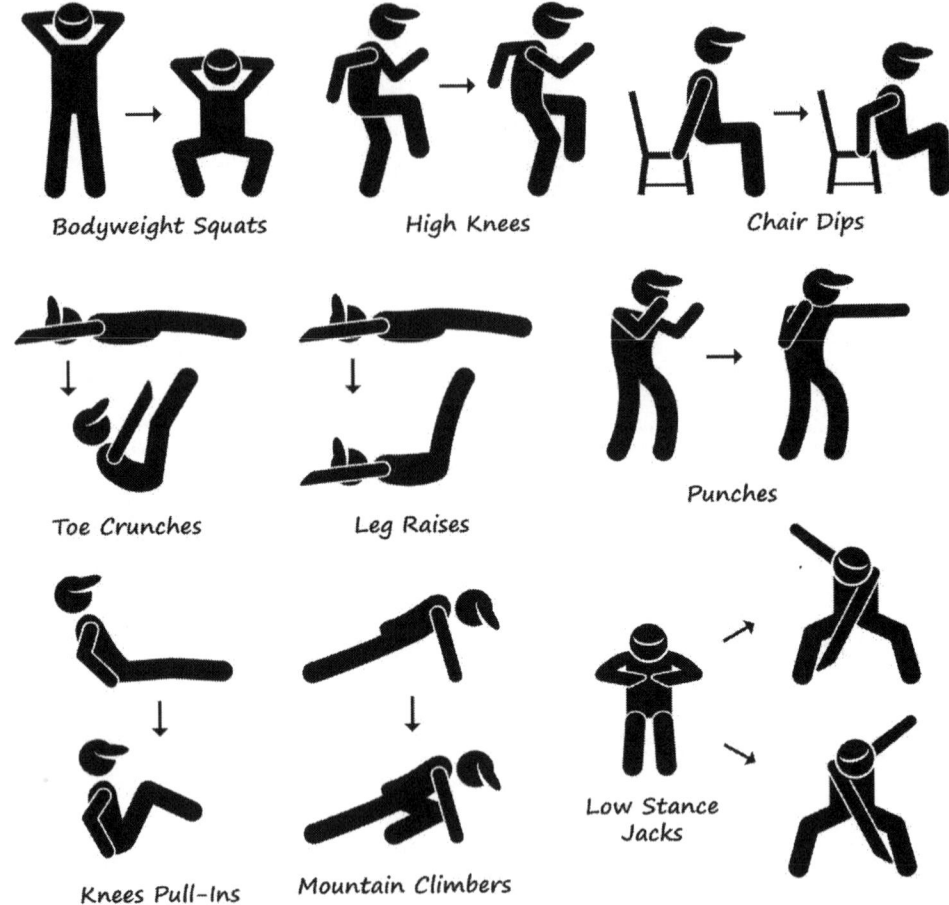

Bodyweight Squats

High Knees

Chair Dips

Toe Crunches

Leg Raises

Punches

Knees Pull-Ins

Mountain Climbers

Low Stance Jacks

I. Full Body

1. Mountain Climbers

Works: abs, upper and lower body, cardiovascular system

Execution:

    a. Go into a forearm plank on the floor with your arms at shoulder width distance.

b. Lift your right foot up to your chest. Repeat with your left foot as though you were climbing a mountain. This is one rep.

c. Do this in a full range of motion.

Variations

    d. Easy

        i. Do the exercise with your palms on a bench.

        ii. Do it slower.

    e. Hard

        iii. Lift your right foot to your left elbow and vice versa.

        iv. Do it faster.

        v. Side mountain climbers

2. Burpees

Works: core, upper and lower body, cardiovascular system

Execution:

    a. Go into a squat and with your hands on your side, plant your palms on the floor.

    b. Kick both your feet back to a strong plank.

    c. Perform a push up.

    d. Jump back up to a squat position and perform an upward jump.

Variations:

    e. Easy

        i. Burpee without push-up: You can just perform a plank instead of a push up.

        ii. Squat thrust: Just stand instead of doing an upward jump.

    f. Hard

        i. Burpee with plank jack: After the push-up, integrate a plank jack by jumping your feet out to your sides (like a jumping jack).

        ii. Long jump-burpee: Instead of jumping upward, jump forward at the end of the movement.

3. Push up

Works: Upper body, core (employs the torso and legs for stability)

Execution:

    a. Go into a plank position with hands on the floor, the distance slightly wider than shoulder width.

    b. Keep your feet together and hold the plank strong.

    c. Keep your body straight: do not arch your back or elevate your butt. Keep your abs tight.

    d. Slowly lower yourself to the ground by bending your elbows at a 90 degree angle.

    e. Push yourself back up until your arms are straightened.

Variations:

    f. Easy

i. Wall push-up: Do a vertical push-up on the wall.
  ii. Knee push-up: Perform a push-up with your knees bent, ankles crossed and feet in the air.
g. Hard
  i. Wide grip push-up: Place your hands wider than shoulder width.
  ii. Single leg or single arm push up: Lift one leg/arm up while doing the push up.
  iii. Diamond push-up: Make a diamond with your hands and perform a push-up.
  iv. Decline push-up: Place your feet on an elevated surface (bench or box).
  v. T-push up: After doing a push-up, raise your left hand upwards. Perform another push-up and raise your right hand upwards.
  vi. Handstand push-up: Slowly walk your legs up the wall to a handstand. Lower yourself slowly and push yourself back up.
  vii. Clapping push-up: As you lift yourself up, clap to come off the floor and go back to the plank position for the next rep.

II. Upper Body

1. Pull up

Works: All upper body muscles

Equipment: a bar that can support your weight (example: monkey bars in the park), door frame or lying under a table (holding on to the table and pulling yourself up to it)

Execution:
  a. Grab the bar with your palms facing away from you.
  b. Hang from the bar with your arms completely straightened.
  c. Try to lift yourself up by using the strength from your arms. Do not swing or jump.
  d. Lift yourself until your chin is in line of the bar.
  e. Slowly lower yourself back down until your arms are completely straightened again.

Variations
  a. Easy
    i. Assisted Pull-up: Have another person to help you lift yourself up. Have him/her hoist you up from the waist.
    ii. Doorknob Pull-up: Place your feet on either side of the door and grab the doorknob. Lean back and bend your knees. Pull your chest up until it touches the door.
  b. Hard
    i. Chest up: Do a pull-up until your chest touches the bar.

iii. Wide grip pull-up: Place your hands on the bar with a slightly wider grip than usual.

2. Isometric Curls
Works: Biceps and forearm
Execution:
   a. Grasp your right wrist with your left hand and put maximum force to push it down.
   b. Attempt to bend at your elbow. Repeat with your other hand.
Variations
   c. Easy
      i. Use half your force.
   d. Hard
      i. Weighted curls: Find a heavy object (bag, milk jug, or a book) and use it as a weight for the bicep curl.

3. Surface Triceps extensions
Works: triceps
Execution:
   a. Find a surface the same height as your waist (bed, table, chair or railing).
   b. Grasp the surface like you're doing an inclined plank/press up, with your hands shoulder-width apart. Step back a little further.
   c. Bend at your elbows and slowly lower your body until your head is just below your hands.
   d. Raise yourself back up to the starting position.
Variations:
   a. Easy
      i. Higher surface triceps extension: Find a higher surface that's the same height as your shoulders or face.
      ii. Side triceps extension: Lie on your side, grab your left shoulder with your right hand and hold your weight with your left shoulder. Lower yourself by bending at your left elbow. Do the same on the other side.
         b. Hard
      iii. Lower surface triceps extension: Find a much lower surface that's the same height as your knees.

4. Dips
Works: triceps (main), chest, shoulders
Equipment: one or two surfaces with the same, waist-high, height (chairs, tables, bed, park bench) that can support your weight
Execution:

a. Grasp both surfaces and raise yourself up until you are supporting your weight with only your arms.
b. With your ankles crossed and your body completely suspended in between the surfaces, slowly lower yourself by bending at your elbows
c. Lift yourself back up.

Variations:
d. Easy
    i. Chair dips: Find a single chair. With your back facing the chair, grasp the surface and straighten your legs in front of you. Slowly lower yourself into a dip.
e. Hard
    ii. One-arm chair dips: Instead of using both hands to support your weight on the chair, use only one.

5. Dive Bombers

Works: Chest, shoulders, triceps
Execution:
a. Assume a plank/press up position and slowly push your butt and back upwards.
b. Swoop chest downwards until it almost touches the ground. Continue the sweeping movement with your shoulders and head until your back is fully arched and you're looking straight ahead.
c. Reverse the movement by doing the sweeping movement using your back until your chest almost touches the ground. Continue this until your butt is back up again.

Variations
f. Easy
    i. Half dive bomber: Do not do the reverse movement. When your chest almost brushes the ground, go back to the starting position.
g. Hard
    i. One leg dive bomber: Use only one leg to support your weight.

III. Core
1. Plank

Works: core muscles
Execution:
a. Place your forearm on the floor with your elbows bent 90 degrees.
b. With your legs together, lift and balance your body. Maintain a straight line.
c. Hold this position for your desired time.

Variations:

a. Easy
ii. Forearm plank: Plant your palms on the ground instead of your elbow.
b. Hard
iii. Up-down plank: To introduce full range of motion to a plank, start with an elbow plank. Plant your right palm then your left on the ground, pushing yourself up. Go back down to an elbow plank and repeat.

2. Sit up
Works: core muscles
Execution:
   a. Lie down on the ground with your knees bent and feet under something that would prevent them from moving, or have another person hold them.
   b. Put your hands behind your head and try to lift yourself up until you feel the contraction. Go back to the starting position and repeat.
Variations:
   c. Easy
      i. Elevated sit up: Place your feet on a low bench, have a partner hold your feet and do a sit up.
   d. Hard
      ii. Weighted sit up: Place a heavy item (book or bag) on your chest and hold it with both your arms while performing a sit up.
      iii. V-up: Lie on the ground with your arms on your sides and your legs together. Lift your legs and shoulders up, balancing only on your butt. Bring your chest and knees towards each other
      iv. Side V-up: Lie on your side with your left hand behind your head and maintain a straight body line. Bend at your hips to bring your left knee to your left elbow. Repeat at the other side.

3. Crunch
Works: abs
Execution:
   h. Lie down on the ground with your knees bent.
   i. With your hands behind your head, roll your shoulders up (just a few inches off the ground) and pull your chest towards your knees until you feel the contraction.
Variations:
   j. Easy
      i. Put your hand on your sides to minimize stress on your neck.

    k. Hard
        i. Bicycle Crunch: While on the ground, lift your bent legs into the air. Put your palms at the back of your head and pull your left leg towards your right elbow and vice versa.

4. Russian Twists

Works: Abs, obliques

Execution:

    l. Lie on the ground and elevate your body to create a V line with your body and your bent legs.

    m. Clasp your stretched hands together and twist your torso your side until your hands are parallel to the floor. Do this in the other side.

Variations:

    n. Hard

        i. Weighted Russian Twists: Use a heavy household item as a weight to carry with both extended hands.

5. Leg Lifts

Works: Lower abs and hips

Execution:

    o. Lie on the ground and place both hands under your butt. Keep your head and shoulders off the floor.

    p. Start with your legs lifted around six inches above the ground and lift your feet until a 45 degree angle to the floor.

    q. Hold this position and slowly lower the legs back to hover six inches from the ground.

13. Variations:

    a. Easy

        i. Single-leg lifts: Lift one leg at a time while the other is rooted to the ground.

        ii. Flutter kicks: Assume starting position of leg lift. Bring one leg up while the other is hovering six inches above. Repeat with the other leg. Do the movement swiftly, like small kicks.

    b. Hard

        i. Hanging bent leg lifts: Suspend your body on a bar, and bring your knees towards your chest.

        ii. Hanging straight leg lifts. While hanging, lift your straight legs up your chest.

IV. Lower Body

1. Squat

Works: quadriceps, glutes, hips, hamstrings

Execution

a. Stand straight with your feet pointing in front and shoulder-width apart.
b. Slowly lower your back and butt while leaning your body forward, until your butt is parallel to the floor.
c. Plant your heels on the ground as you stand back up.

Variations

d. Easy
   i. Half-squats: Decrease the depth of your squat to half.
   ii. Air squats: Do squats with your arms in front of you.
   iii. Prisoner squats: Do squats with your hands at the back of your head.
   iv. Wall sit: Rest your back on a wall and squat for a desired number of minutes.
e. Hard
   i. Sumo squat: Do a squat with a wide stance on your legs, a larger angle than the classic squat. Your toes should face slightly out.
   ii. One-legged squat: Find a surface that you can hold on to while doing a squat with one leg raised and the other supporting your weight.
   iii. Pistol squat: Lift one leg up and balance with your other as you bring your butt lower to the ground.

2. Box Jumps

Works: quadriceps, glutes, hamstrings, lower back, calves
Equipment: Box/ Stairs/ sturdy chair
Execution:

a. Find a stable surface that you can jump on.
b. Start with a half squat to gain momentum and jump on the surface. The higher the surface, the harder the exercise.
c. Jump variations:
   a. Easy
   b. Jump Squat: Squat then explode to a jump. Land back into a squat and repeat.
   c. Lateral Jump: Jump explosively from side to side.
d. Hard
   a. Star jumpers: Do a wide angled sumo squat starting position with your palms on the floor. Jump explosively with your arms and legs stretched out. Land back to the starting position.

3. Lunge

Works: quadriceps and glutes
a. Execution:

a. Stand straight and take a big step forward with your right leg, bending your left knees until it almost touches the floor. Both knees should be in a 90 degree angle.
b. Repeat on the other leg.
b. Variations:
a. Easy
a. Back Lunges: Take a step backward instead of forward.
b. Side Lunges: Stand straight with your hands in front of your legs. Take a large step to the right and shift your weight towards that side. Do the same on the other leg.
c. Hard
i. Walking Lunge: Lunges while walking
ii. Walking Lunge with kickback: Do walking lunges and kick the back leg back
iii. Jumping lunges: Start with the bent-knees position of the classic lunge and push your front foot into a jump. Switch legs while on air and land on the other leg back to a bent knees position.
iv. Lunge with Russian twist: Lunge and twist at the end of the movement

Chapter 6

Workout Routines You May Want to Try

BEGINNERS WORK OUT			
Warm up: 5-10 minutes dynamic stretching Cool down: Light jog then stretching			
Day	Week 1 (3 x 12 reps)	Week 2 (3 x 12 reps)	Week 3 (3 x 12-15 reps)	Week 4 (3 x 12-15 reps)
Day 1 (Full body)	1.Jumping Rope (3x50 reps) 2. Squat 3. Wall Push-up 4. Forward lunge 5. Step ups (box, stairs or chair) 6. Chair Dips	1. Jumping Jacks (3x50 reps) 2. Air squat 3. Knee Push-up 4. Walking Forward Lunge 5. Step ups (box, stairs or chair) 6. Chair dips	1.Tuck Jump 2. Prisoner squat 3. Knee Push-up 4. Walking forward lunge 5. Box jump 6. Bar/surface dips 7. Russian Twists	1. Tuck Jump 2. Prisoner Squat (as low as you can) 3. Push-up 4. Walking forward lunge with kick 5. Box jump 6.Surface dips 7. Russian Twists
Day 2 (Upper Body)	1. Squat Thrust 2.Wall Push-up 3. Side triceps extensions 4. Chair dips 5. Door frame or table pull up	1. Squat Thrust 2. Knee Push-up 3. Side triceps extensions 4. Chair dips 5. Door-frame or table pull up	1. Burpees 2. Knee Push-up 3.Surface triceps extensions 4. Surface dips (two chairs/tables) 5. Door-fame or table pull up 6. Half dive bomber	1. Burpees 2. Push-up 3.Surface triceps extensions 4. Surface dips (two chairs/tables) 5. Door-frame or table pull up 6. Half dive bomber
Day 3	Active recovery Light Aerobic Activity/ Stretching/ Yoga			
Day 4 (Core)	1. Forearm Plank (15 seconds) 2. Elevated Sit up 3. Crunches with hands on the side 4. Plank Jack 5. Russian Twist	1.Elbow Plank (15 seconds) 2. Elevated Sit up 3. Crunches 4. Plank Jack 5. Russian Twist 6. Single Leg Lifts	1.Elbow Plank (30 seconds) 2. Sit ups 3. Crunches 4. Plank Jack 5. Russian Twist 6. Single Leg Lifts	1.Elbow Plank (30 seconds) 2. Sit ups 3. Crunches 4. Plank Jack 5. Russian Twist 6. Flutter Kicks
Day 5 (Lower Body)	1.Half squat 2. Wall sit (15 seconds) 3. Lateral Jump 4. Forward Lunge 5. Step up on a knee-high surface	1.Squat 2. Wall sit (15 seconds) 3. Box Jump 4. Forward Lunge 5. Step up on a knee-high surface	1.Squat 2. Wall sit (30 seconds) 3. Box Jump 4. Forward Lunge 5. Steps on stairs (1 minute)	1.Squat 2. Wall sit (30 seconds) 3. Box Jump 4. Forward Lunge 5. Backward Lunge 6. Steps on stairs

	(one leg at a time)	(one leg at a time)	6. Squat Jump	(1 minute) 7. Squat Jump
Day 6 (Full Body)	1.Jumping Rope (3x50 reps) 2. Squat 3. Wall Push-up 4. Forward lunge 5. Step ups (box or chair) 6. Chair Dips	1. Jumping Jacks (3x50 reps) 2. Air squat 3. Knee Push-up 4. Walking Forward Lunge 5. Step ups (box or chair) 6. Chair dips	1.Tuck Jump 2. Prisoner squat 3. Knee Push-up 4. Walking forward lunge 5. Box jump 6. Bar/surface dips 7. Russian Twists	1. Tuck Jump 2. Prisoner Squat (as low as you can) 3. Push-up 4. Walking forward lunge with kick 5. Box jump 6.Surface dips 7. Russian Twists
Day 7	Active recovery Light Aerobic Activity/ Stretching/ Yoga			

INTERMEDIATE WORK OUT

Warm up: 5-10 minutes dynamic stretching
Cool down: Light jog then stretching

Day	Week 1 (3 x 12 reps, 15 seconds rest)	Week 2 (3 x 12 reps, 15 seconds rest)	Week 3 (3 x 12-15 reps, 10 seconds rest)	Week 4 (3 x 12-15 reps, 10 seconds rest)
Day 1 (Full body)	1. Mountain climbers 2. Squat 3. Push-up 4. Walking Forward lunge 5. Box Jump 6. Surface Dips 7. Burpees without push-up	1. Mountain climbers 2. Sumo squat 3. Push-up 4. Walking Forward Lunge 5. Box Jump 6. Surface Dips 7. Burpees without push-up	1. Mountain climbers (fast) 2. Jump squat 3. Push-up 4. Walking lunge with kickback 5. Box jump 6. Bar/surface dips 7. Burpees	1. Mountain climbers (fast) 2. Jump squat 3. T Push-up 4. Tuck jump 5. Walking lunge with kickback 6. Box jump 7. Bar/surface dips 8. Burpees
Day 2 (Upper Body)	1. Bar pull up 2. Wide Grip Push-up 3. Push up 4. Side triceps extensions 5. Surface dips 6. Weighted Curls 7. Half dive bomber	1. Bar pull up 2. Wide Grip Push-up 3. Decline Push-up 4. Surface triceps extensions 5. Surface dips 6. Weighted Curls 7. Dive bomber	1. Bar pull up 2. T-push up 3. Decline Push-up 4. Surface triceps extensions 5. Burpees 6. Surface dips 7. Weighted Curls 8. Dive bomber	1. Wide grip pull up 2. T-push up 3. Decline Push-up 4. Surface triceps extensions 5. Burpees 6. Surface dips (with weight ex: bag) 7. Weighted Curls 8. Dive bomber
Day 3	Active recovery Light Aerobic Activity/ Stretching/ Yoga			
Day 4 (Core)	1. Elbow Plank (45 seconds) 2. Sit up 3. Crunches 4. Plank Jack 5. Russian Twist 6. Single leg lifts	1. Elbow Plank (45 seconds) 2. Sit up 3. Crunches 4. Plank Jack 5. Russian Twist 6. Leg Lifts	1. Elbow Plank (50 seconds) 2. Sit up 3. Crunches 4. Bicycle crunches 5. Up-down plank 6. Weighted Russian Twist 7. Leg Lifts	1. Elbow Plank (1 minute) 2. Sit ups 3. Crunches 4. Bicycle crunches 5. Up-down plank 6. Weighted Russian Twist 7. Flutter Kicks
Day 5 (Lower Body)	1. Sumo squat 2. Prisoner squat 3. Jump Squat 4. Walking lunge	1. Sumo squat 2. Prisoner squat 3. Jump Squat 4. Back lunge	1. One-legged squat 2. Sumo squat 3. Jump Squat	1. One-legged squat 2. Sumo squat 3. Jump Squat

	with kickback 5. Box jump 6. Wall sit (45 seconds)	5. Lunge with Russian twist 6. Box jump 7. Wall sit (45 seconds)	4. Back lunge 5. Walking lunge with Russian twist 6. Jumping lunges 7. Box jump 8. Wall sit (45 seconds)	4. Back lunge 5. Walking lunge with Russian twist 6. Jumping lunges 7. Box jump 8. Wall sit (1 minute)
Day 6 (Full Body)	1.Mountain climbers 2. Squat 3. Push-up 4. Walking Forward lunge 5. Box Jump 6. Surface Dips 7. Burpees without push-up	1. Mountain climbers 2. Sumo squat 3. Push-up 4. Walking Forward Lunge 5. Box Jump 6.Surface Dips 7. Burpees without push-up	1. Mountain climbers (fast) 2. Jump squat 3. Push-up 4. Walking lunge with kickback 5. Box jump 6. Bar/surface dips 7. Burpees	1. Mountain climbers (fast) 2. Jump squat 3. T Push-up 4. Tuck jump 5. Walking lunge with kickback 6. Box jump 7. Bar/surface dips 8. Burpees
Day 7 (Full Body)	Active recovery Light Aerobic Activity/ Stretching/ Yoga			

ADVANCED WORK OUT

Warm up: 5-10 minutes dynamic stretching
Cool down: Light jog then stretching

Day	Week 1 (4 x 12 reps, 15 seconds rest)	Week 2 (4 x 12 reps, 15 seconds rest)	Week 3 (4 x 12-15 reps, 10 seconds rest)	Week 4 (4 x 15 reps, 10 seconds rest)
Day 1 (Full body)	1. Burpee with plank jack 2. Mountain Climbers 3. T push up 4. Jumping Lunge 5. Jump Squat 6. Surface Dips 7. Pull up	1. Burpee with plank jack 2. Mountain Climbers (fast) 3. T Push-up 4. Jumping lunge 5. Box Jump 6. Surface Dips 7. Wide grip pull up 8. Dive Bomber	1. Long-jump burpee 2. Mountain Climbers (fast) 3. T Push-up 4. Up-down plank 5. Jumping lunge 6. Box Jump 7. Surface Dips 8. Wide grip pull up 9. Dive Bomber	1. Long jump burpee 2. Mountain Climbers (fast) 3. T Push-up 4. Up-down plank 5. Jumping lunge 6. Box Jump 7. V-up 8. Surface Dips 9. Wide grip pull up 10. Dive Bomber
Day 2 (Upper Body)	1. Pull up 2. Chest up 3. Wide Grip Push-up 4. Diamond Push up 5. T-push up 6. Side triceps extensions (hold 3 seconds in mid-extension) 7. Surface dips 8. One-arm chair dips	1. Pull up 2. Chest up 3. Diamond Push-up 4. T push up 5. Handstand push up 6. Lower surface triceps extensions (hold 5 seconds in mid-extension) 7. Surface dips 8. One-arm chair dips 9. Dive bombers	1. Pull up 2. Chest up 3. Diamond Push-up 4. T push up 5. Handstand push up 6. Side triceps extensions (hold 8 seconds in mid-extension) 7. Surface dips 8. One-arm chair dips 9. One leg dive bombers 10. One arm push-up	1. Pull up 2. Chest up 3. Diamond Push-up 4. T push up 5. Handstand push up 6. Clapping push up 7. Lower surface triceps extensions (hold 10 seconds in mid-extension) 8. Surface dips (prolong movement for 5 seconds) 9. One-arm chair dips 10. One leg dive bombers 11. One arm push-up
Day 3	Active recovery Light Aerobic Activity/ Stretching/ Yoga			
Day 4 (Core)	1. Elbow Plank (1 minute) 2. Weighted Sit up	1. Elbow Plank (1 minute) 2. Weighted Sit up	1. Elbow Plank (1 minute, 15 seconds)	1. Elbow Plank (1 minute, 30 seconds)

	3. Crunches 4. Bicycle Crunches 5. Forearm Plank (1 minute) 6. Weighted Russian Twist 7. Hanging bent leg lifts 8. V-up	3. Crunches 4. Bicycle Crunches 5. Forearm Plank (1 minute) 6. Up-down plank 7. Side V-up 8. Weighted Russian Twist 9. Hanging bent leg lifts 10. V-up	2. Weighted Sit up 3. Crunches 4. Bicycle Crunches 5. Forearm Plank (1 minute, 15 seconds) 6. Up-down plank 7. Side V-up 8. Weighted Russian Twist 9. Hanging straight leg lifts 10. V-up	2. Weighted Sit up 3. Crunches 4. Bicycle Crunches 5. Forearm Plank (1 minute, 15 seconds) 6. Up-down plank 7. Side V-up 8. Weighted Russian Twist 9. Hanging straight leg lifts (hold for 5 seconds) 10. V-up
Day 5 (Lower Body)	1. Jump squat 2. Pistol Squat 3. Long Jump Burpee 4. Lunge with Russian Twist 5. Jumping Lunge 6. High Box jump 7. Wall sit (1 minute)	1. Jump squat 2. Star jumpers 3. Pistol squat 4. Long jump burpee 5. Jumping Lunge with Russian Twist 6. Walking Lunge with kickback 7. High box jump 8. Wall sit (1 minute, 30 seconds)	1. Jump squat (lowest squat, highest jump) 2. Star jumpers 3. Pistol squat 4. Long jump burpee 5. Jumping Lunge with Russian Twist 6. Back lunge 7. Walking lunge with kickback 8. High box jump 9. Wall sit (2 minutes) 10. Burpee with plank jack	1. Jump squat (lowest squat, highest jump) 2. Star jumpers 3. Pistol squat (hold for 5 seconds) 4. Long jump burpee 5. Jumping Lunge with Russian Twist 6. Back lunge 7. Walking lunge with kickback 8. High box jump 9. Wall sit (2 minutes 30 seconds) 10. Burpee with plank jack
Day 6 (Full Body)	1. Burpee with plank jack 2. Mountain Climbers 3. T push up 4. Jumping Lunge 5. Jump Squat 6. Surface Dips	1. Burpee with plank jack 2. Mountain Climbers (fast) 3. T Push-up 4. Jumping lunge 5. Box Jump 6. Surface Dips	1. Long-jump burpee 2. Mountain Climbers (fast) 3. T Push-up 4. Up-down plank 5. Jumping lunge 6. Box Jump	1. Long jump burpee 2. Mountain Climbers (fast) 3. T Push-up 4. Up-down plank 5. Jumping lunge 6. Box Jump

	7. Pull up	7. Wide grip pull up 8. Dive Bomber	7.Surface Dips 8. Wide grip pull up 9. Dive Bomber	7.V-up 8.Surface Dips 9. Wide grip pull up 10. Dive Bomber
Day 7 (Full Body)	Active recovery Light Aerobic Activity/ Stretching/ Yoga			

Conclusion

I hope you have enjoyed this book and the simple steps presented in it to help you get motivated, fit and healthy through healthy eating and bodyweight workouts.

Thank you again for downloading this book, I hope it has inspired you to take action even if only small steps to reach your health, and fitness goals.

Through the chapters above you will have discovered how having clear goals, visioning what the end result looks like, ensuring you have a positive mindset, and then taking action will lead you to achieving your goals in the short, medium and long term.

Remember it is the long term trend that is your friend, as you work over the long term on all the areas covered in this book you will begin to see your goals come into site, whether it be feelings of hope through positive mental practices, weight loss or increasing strength or fitness all these take time and commitment.

With a commitment to taking action you will begin to see a small but growing positive change in your health and fitness.

I wish you every success as you continue to strive towards your health and fitness goals and go from strength to strength. Although with a positive mental attitude and commitment action you wont need any luck as it will be you that achieves these goals through your own hard work.

Thanks again and enjoy your newfound health and fitness.

Quick start up guide

- Set a clear goal, define 3-5 the steps to get there, when, what, how and why you will and want to achieve it.
- Right down and read out load positive motivating statements about this goal.
- Address your barriers (or excuses) so that when they arise you already have answers for them
- Visualize yourself achieving the steps and ultimate goal

- Measure where you are now and track your progress.
- Reward yourself for even small successes.

Eat less and better

- Eat from smaller plates and measure out your food
- Have a glass of water before eating. In fact drink water often its good for you.
- Carry healthy snacks around with you throughout the day to prevent cravings
- Make simple home cooked food with fresh produce including fruits, vegetables, whole grain products, and eat more of these.
- Eat less sweets, biscuit/cookies, sugary drinks and fast food as they aren't doing you any good.

Bodyweight workouts

- Make sure your workout starts with a warm up exercise, which can obviously be part of the work out i.e. star jumps. And end with a cool down exercise
- You can tweak the exercises for your own goals, whether fitness, strength, flexibility, balance or coordination.
-

Quick 10 minute work out

 min star jumps

 min opposite knew to elbow
 minute plank
 min press ups
 min squats
 minute Russian twist
 min sit ups
 min mountain climbers
 min burpees
 min opposite knee to elbow
Rest

I Need Your Help…

Thank you for downloading the book! I hope you enjoyed it and found it informative and entertaining.

If you enjoyed this book, then I'd like to ask you for a favor? Could you be so kind to leave an honest review for the book on Amazon? It'd greatly appreciate it!

>>Click here to leave an honest review on Amazon.com<<

I want to reach as many people as I can with this book, and more reviews will help me accomplish that.

Thank you for your time and best wishes to you and your fitness journey!

About the Author

Hello my name is Rob James and this is my book.

I am about average height, according to my scales often a little overweight but have always been keen to keen to get fit and healthy. Occasionally I have wanted to be a particular weight and every summer to feel comfortable when at the pool or beachside. However I have struggled to match these desires with action. I guess life just happened to me.

Recently I began to look at people who had achieved their goals or were close to them and thought how did they do that. Well to boil it down to one sentence, they came up with and plan and then took action.

So I now try and come up with plans for nearly everything, finances, a happy marriage and getting fit amongst many things.

I hope through what I have learnt and presented in this book it will help you combine the areas of simple nutrition, positive mental attitude and easily actionable bodyweight workouts to achieve your health and fitness goals.

Printed in Great Britain
by Amazon

57992338R00037